Operation Primer

LAPAROSCOPIC SIGMOIDECTOMY FOR DIVERTICULITIS

Editors

Marc Immenroth
Thorsten Berg
Jürgen Brenner

Authors

Hans-Peter Bruch
Uwe Johannes Roblick
Hamed Esnaashari

assisted by

Ann-Katrin Güler
Ute Stefani Haaga

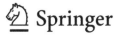 Springer

Authors

Hans-Peter Bruch, M.D., PhD
Director of the Surgical Department, University of Schleswig-Holstein, Campus Lübeck,
Ratzeburger Allee 160, 23538 Lübeck, Germany

Uwe Johannes Roblick, M.D., PhD
Vice Director of the Surgical Department, University of Schleswig-Holstein, Campus Lübeck,
Ratzeburger Allee 160, 23538 Lübeck, Germany

Hamed Esnaashari, M.D.
Surgical Department, University of Schleswig-Holstein, Campus Lübeck,
Ratzeburger Allee 160, 23538 Lübeck, Germany

Editors

Marc Immenroth, PhD
European Clinical Studies Manager, Ethicon Endo-Surgery (Europe) GmbH,
Hummelsbütteler Steindamm 71, 22851 Norderstedt, Germany

Thorsten Berg, M.D.
Senior Manager Health Outcome, Ethicon Endo-Surgery (Europe) GmbH,
Hummelsbütteler Steindamm 71, 22851 Norderstedt, Germany

Jürgen Brenner, M.D.
Managing Director, Ethicon Endo-Surgery Germany (Johnson & Johnson MEDICAL GmbH),
Hummelsbütteler Steindamm 71, 22851 Norderstedt, Germany

ISBN 978-3-540-78451-7   Laparoscopic Sigmoidectomy for Diverticulitis

Bibliografische Information der Deutschen Bibliothek
The Deutsche Bibliothek lists this publication in Deutsche Nationalbibliographie;
detailed bibliographic data is available in the internet at http://dnb.ddb.de.

First published in Germany in 2008 by Springer Medizin Verlag
springer.com

© Ethicon Endo-Surgery (Europe) GmbH

SPIN 12235018
Layout and typesetting: Dr. Carl GmbH, Stuttgart, Germany
Printing: Stürtz GmbH, Würzburg, Germany

18/5135/DK – 5 4 3 2 1 0

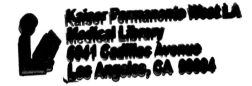

This book has been sponsored by Ethicon Endo-Surgery (Europe) GmbH and Johnson & Johnson MEDICAL GmbH, Norderstedt, Germany. The authors are responsible for the content of the publication. Information provided in this book is offered in good faith as an educational tool for health care professionals. The information has been thoroughly reviewed and is believed to be useful and accurate at the time of its publication, but is offered without warranty of any kind. The authors and the sponsors shall not be responsible for any loss or damage arising from its use.

Editors' preface

The idea for the Operation Primer originated in a scientific study entitled "Mental Training in Surgical Education" that formed part of a collaborative project between the surgical department of the University of Cologne, the Institute of Sports and Sport Sciences of the University of Heidelberg and the European Surgical Institute (ESI) in Norderstedt.

The aim of the study was to evaluate the effect of mental training, which has been used successfully in top-class sports for decades, on surgical training. However, in order for mental training to be applied to surgery, it first had to undergo modification. In the course of this modification, the first Operation Primer was produced, the layout of which was largely adopted for the final version presented here.

Over several years the design of the Operation Primer was optimized and applied to other operations. At the same time, a team of authors was found who could transform the concept into a series of practical surgical primers. For this Operation Primer our first and very special thanks go to the authors Hans-Peter Bruch, Uwe Johannes Roblick and Hamed Esnaashari, without whom it would not have been possible even to begin to think of converting our ideas into reality.

The text of the Operation Primer is fully comprehendible only when used in conjunction with the accompanying photographs. We would like to thank the Karl Storz Company who provided the camera and technical expertise for most of the pictures featured in the Operation Primer. A number of photographs were also provided by Dr. Robert Keller.

Reality often requires an abstraction in order to make certain situations clearer. This was the reason for including line drawings throughout the Operation Primer. These diagrams were produced by Thomas Heller, whom we gratefully acknowledge.

Our concept of practical surgical primers will become a reality through Dr. Carl GmbH and Springer Medizin Verlag Heidelberg.

The Operation Primers will be produced with the aim of describing the various operations in the simplest possible manner, but without over-simplifying. Although most time has been spent on the establishment of the scientific basis behind the operations the main focus has always been on the practical relevance of the Primers.

With this Operation Primer we hope we have met our own as well as the readers' highest expectations.

The Editors   March 2008

Authors' preface

In past several years laparoscopic methods have gained widespread use in visceral surgery and a wealth of experience has been gained. The vision of the laparoscopic pioneers, foreseeing the potential impact of laparoscopy in colorectal surgery, deserves high credit. The changes following this development produced a variety of new techniques for the entire surgical team. This knowledge had to be stratified and finally to be disseminated. The Operation Primer Laparoscopic Sigmoidectomy for Diverticulitis gives a detailed overview of the patients' preparation, key operation steps, postoperative care, and pitfalls of the operation. The major goal was to provide a comprehensive handbook for laparoscopic colorectal surgeons, helping to avoid those pitfalls that lead to complications. The operational steps described represent the technique used in Lübeck where more than 2000 laparoscopic colorectal resections of different kinds have been performed. The authors hope that the Operation Primer will be of great use to both the novice and the advanced laparoscopic colorectal surgeon.

Hans-Peter Bruch
Uwe Johannes Roblick
Hamed Esnaashari

March 2008

Editors

Marc Immenroth, PhD

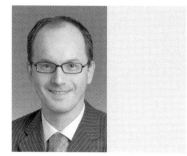

- Studied Psychology (Diploma) and Sports Science (Master) in Heidelberg, Germany
- 1999–2006 Sport-Psychologist (including consultant to many German top athletes during their preparation for the World-Championships and Olympics) and Industrial Psychologist (including consultant to Lufthansa Inc.)
- 2000 Research Scientist at the University of Greifswald, Germany (Policlinic for Restorative Dentistry and Periodontology)
- 2001–2004 Research Scientist at the University of Heidelberg, Germany (Institute for Sports and Sports Science)
- 2002 Doctorate in Psychology at the University of Heidelberg, Germany
- 2005–2006 Assistant Lecturer at the University of Giessen, Germany (Institute of Sport)
- 2006–2008 Assistant Professor at the University of Greifswald, Germany (Institute of Sport)
- Since 2006 European Clinical Studies Manager at Ethicon Endo-Surgery Europe in Norderstedt, Germany

Focus of Research and Work
- Mental Training in Sport, Surgery and Aviation
- Virtual Reality in Surgical Education
- Coping with Emotion and Stress

Author of many scientific articles and textbooks in psychology, sports science and medicine

Thorsten Berg, M.D.

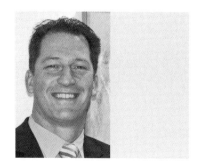

- Studied Medicine in Heidelberg, Germany
- 1996 Intern at the University Hospital, Durban, South Africa
- 1997 Intern at the Surgical Department of the General Hospital, Ludwigshafen, Germany
- 2003 Qualified as General Surgeon
- 2003 Director of Education of European Surgical Institute in Norderstedt, Germany
- 2005 Director of Clinical Development at Ethicon Endo-Surgery Europe in Norderstedt, Germany
- Since 2006 Senior Manager Health Outcome at Ethicon Endo-Surgery Europe in Norderstedt, Germany
- 2007 Doctorate in Medicine at the University of Heidelberg, Germany

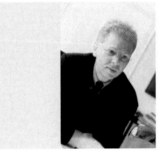

Jürgen Brenner, M.D.

- Studied Medicine in Hamburg, Germany
- 1972 Medical Doctor at University of Hamburg, Germany
- 1972 Institute for Neuroanatomy, University of Hamburg, Germany
- 1974 Senior Resident at the Department of Surgery of the General Hospital Hamburg-Wandsbek, Germany
- 1981 Medical Director of Department for Colorectal and Trauma Surgery at St. Adolf Stift Hospital in Reinbek, Germany
- 1987 Director for Surgical Research of Ethicon Inc. in Norderstedt, Germany
- 1989 Director of European Surgical Institute and Vice President Professional Education Europe of Ethicon Endo-Surgery Europe in Norderstedt, Germany
- Since 2004 Managing Director Ethicon Endo-Surgery Germany in Norderstedt, Germany

Assistants

Ann-Katrin Güler

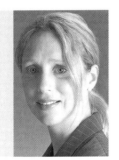

- Studied Medicine in Hamburg, Germany
- Since 2005 doctoral thesis 'Development and evaluation of standardized operation primer for education in minimal invasive surgery' at the University of Hamburg, Germany (Department of General, Thoracic and Visceral Surgery)
- Since 2007 member of the Market Access department at Ethicon Endo-Surgery Europe in Norderstedt, Germany

Ute Stefani Haaga, M.D.

- Studied Medicine in Freiburg, Germany
- 2000–2002 Intern at the Department of Medicine at the University of Erlangen, Germany
- 2001 Doctorate in Medicine at the University of Freiburg, Germany
- Since 2002 Project Manager and Medical Writer at Dr. Carl GmbH in Stuttgart, Germany

Authors

Hans-Peter Bruch, M.D.

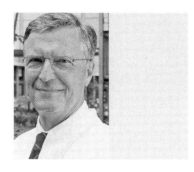

- Studied Medicine in Würzburg, Hamburg and Munich, Germany
- 1970 Academic studies at the Protein Institute in Munich, Germany
- 1970–1972 DFG Research Grant for Biochemistry: Biochemical Institute
  Würzburg, Germany
- 1975 Surgical internship at the Surgical Department, University of Würzburg,
  Germany
- 1980 Von Langenbeck Research Award of the German Surgical Society (DGCH)
- 1981 Specialist in General Surgery
- 1981 Thesis of postdoctoral lecture qualification
- 1982 Appointment as a University Professor
- 1982 Assistant Medical Director at the Surgical Department, University of
  Würzburg, Germany
- 1986 Specialist in Vascular Surgery
- 1988 Consultant Surgeon of the German Armed Forces
- Since 1990 Director of the Surgical Department, University of Lübeck, Germany
- Since 1996 Specialist in Visceral Surgery
- 1996 Head of the working group "Coloproctology of the German Society of
  Surgeons"
- 1996 Western Europe Representative of the ISUCRS (International Society of
  University Colon and Rectal Surgeons)
- 1997 Member of the Board of the North Western German Surgical Society
- 1999 Member of the Leopoldina
- 2003 Spokesman of the German Convent of University Visceral Surgeons
- 2004–2007 Secretary of the German Society of Visceral Surgery
- 2007 Incoming president of the German Society of General and Visceral Surgery

Member of various editorial boards, co-editor and editor of several surgical journals.

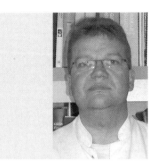

Uwe Johannes Roblick, M.D., PhD

- Studied Medicine in Würzburg, Germany
- 1994–1995 Intern at the Department of Surgery, Juliusspital Würzburg, Germany
- Doctorate in Medicine at the University of Würzburg, Germany
- 1995 Intern at the Department of Surgery, University of Schleswig-Holstein, Campus Lübeck, Germany
- 2001 Specialist in General Surgery at the Department of Surgery, University of Schleswig-Holstein, Campus Lübeck, Germany
- 2002 Adolf Kußmaul Research Award
- 2003 Specialist surgeon at the Department of Surgery, Akademiska Sjukhuset, Uppsala University, Sweden
- 2004 Doctorate in Molecular Oncology at the Karolinska Institute, Stockholm, Sweden
- Since 2005 Vice Director at the Department of Surgery, University of Schleswig-Holstein, Campus Lübeck, Germany
- 2006 Von Langenbeck Research Award of the German Surgical Society (DGCH)

Focus of Research and Work
- Coordinator of the CHIR-NET study center, Lübeck, Germany

Author of more than 100 scientific publications

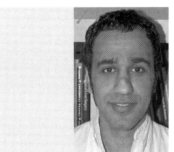

Hamed Esnaashari, M.D.

- Studied Medicine at the University of Lübeck, Germany
- Since 2003 Intern at the Department of Surgery, University of Schleswig-Holstein, Campus Lübeck, Germany
- Doctorate in Medicine at the University of Schleswig Holstein, Lübeck, Germany

The authors gratefully acknowledge the assistance of Robert Keller, M.D., Department of Surgery, University of Schleswig-Holstein, Campus Lübeck, Germany.

Contents

V Management of difficult situations, complications and mistakes

VI Anatomical variations

Appendix

Introduction

From an educational point of view, the Operation Primer is somewhat plagiaristic. The layout – and this can be admitted freely – is largely taken over from commonly available cook books. In such books, the ingredients and cooking utensils required to prepare the recipe in question are normally listed first. The most important cooking procedures are then described briefly in the text. Photographs support the written explanations and show what the dish should look like when prepared. Sometimes diagrams and illustrations make individual cooking steps clearer.

Despite these obvious parallels, there is a crucial difference between cook books and the Operation Primer: in the Operation Primer, complicated and complex surgical techniques are described that are intended to help the surgeon and his team perform an operation safely and economically. Ultimately, it always comes down to the patient's welfare. The following must therefore be said early in this introduction:

• The use of the Operation Primer as an aid to operating requires that conventional and minimally invasive techniques have first been completely mastered.

• Being alert to possible mistakes is categorically the most important principle when operating. It applies to an even greater extent to minimally invasive surgery than it does to conventional surgery; avoiding mistakes is crucial.

As already mentioned in the foreword, the concept of the Operation Primer originated in a scientific study with the title "Mental Training in Surgical Education" that formed part of a collaborative project between the surgical department of the University of Cologne (under Prof. Hans Troidl), the Institute of Sports and Sport Science of the University of Heidelberg and the European Surgical Institute (ESI) in Norderstedt. Laparoscopic cholecystectomy was the initial focus.

Mental training is derived from top-class sports. This is understood as the methodically repeated and conscious imagination of actions and movements without actually carrying them out at the same time (cf. Driskell, Copper & Moran, 1994; Eberspächer, 2001; Feltz & Landers, 1983; Immenroth, 2003). Scientific involvement with imagining movement has a long tradition in medical and psychological research. As early as 1852, Lotze described how imagining and perceiving movements can lead to a concurrent performance "with quiet movements …" (Lotze, 1852). This phenomenon later became known by the names "Ideomotion" and "Carpenter effect" (Carpenter, 1874).

In the collaborative project, mental training was modified in such a way that it could be employed in the training and further education of young surgeons. In mental training in surgery, the surgeon imagines the operation from the inner perspective without performing any actual movements, i.e. he goes through the operation step by step in his mind's eye. In the study that was conducted at the European Surgical Institute (ESI), the first Operation Primer was used as the basis for this imagination. In this primer, laparoscopic cholecystectomy was subdivided into individual, clearly depicted steps, the so-called nodal points.

The study evaluated the effect of the mental training on learning laparoscopic cholecystectomy compared with practical training and with a control group. The planning, conducting and evaluation of the study took 7 years (2000–2007), with over 100 surgeons participating.

The results corresponded exactly with the expectations: the mentally trained surgeons improved in a similar degree to those surgeons who received additional practical training on a pelvi trainer simulator (in some subscales even more). Moreover, there was greater improvement in these two groups compared with the control group, which did not receive any additional mental or practical training (cf. in detail, Immenroth, Bürger, Brenner, Nagelschmidt, Eberspächer & Troidl, 2007; Immenroth, Bürger, Brenner, Kemmler, Nagelschmidt, Eberspächer & Troidl, 2005; Immenroth, Eberspächer, Nagelschmidt, Troidl, Bürger, Brenner, Berg, Müller & Kemmler, 2005).

Furthermore, the study included a questionnaire to determine the extent to which the mentally trained surgeons accepted mental training as a teaching method in surgery. Mental training was assessed as very positive by all 34 mentally trained surgeons. The Operation Primer received particular acclaim in the evaluation (cf. in detail, Immenroth et al., 2007):

- 28 surgeons wished to use similar self-made Operation Primers in their daily work.

- 29 surgeons attributed the success of the mental training at least in part to the Operation Primer.

- 30 surgeons wanted to have these Operation Primers as a fixed component of the course at the European Surgical Institute (ESI).

This positive response to the study was the starting point for the production of the present series of Operation Primers.

Before publication, the Operation Primer was developed by methodical and didactical means and then adapted to the readers' needs and wishes. This was carried out after a survey of 93 surgeons (interns, resident doctors, assistant medical directors and medical directors), who participated in surgical courses at the European Surgical Institute (ESI). They evaluated in detail the structure and components by means of a questionnaire.

The results of this survey gave important findings on how to optimize the Operation Primer. The sense and representation of the nodal points, the comprehensibility and detail of the text, and the photographs of the operation were highly valued especially by young surgeons (Güler, Immenroth, Berg, Bürger & Gawad, 2006). The comprehensive research undertaken with this Operation Primer series will ensure its overall value to the reader.

Structure and handling of the Operation Primer

In the present series of Operation Primers, an attempt has been made to standardize the described laparoscopic operations as much as possible. This is achieved on the one hand by applying the same structure to all operational techniques described. On the other hand, operative sequences that are performed identically in all operations are always explained by using the same blocks of text. By following a general structure for the description of all operations and by using identical text blocks, it was intended to aid recognition of recurring patterns and their translation into action even for different operations.

The Operation Primer is divided into six chapters, each identified by Roman numerals and different register colors on the margin. This structure applies to all the Operation Primers in the present series. The contents of the individual chapters will now be explained.

In **Preparations for the operation,** the basic instruments for all laparoscopic operations and then the additional laparoscopic instruments for the specific operation are listed. This is followed by a detailed description of the positioning and shaving of the patient, attaching the neutral electrode, setting the equipment, skin disinfection and sterile draping of the patient. The operative preparation is concluded with a detailed description and picture of how the operating team is to be positioned for the operation in question.

In the chapter **Creating the pneumoperitoneum – placing the optical trocar,** three alternatives are shown in detail: the Hasson method, trocar with optical obturator, and Veress needle. The choice of method is up to the individual surgeon. All three alternatives are employed in surgical practice. However, it should be pointed out that the greatest danger in minimally invasive surgery is the insertion of the Veress needle as it is done "blind".

Placing the working trocars is explained in detail in the next chapter. The written explanations are supplemented by diagrams. In order to keep a constant overview of the placement of the trocars, even during the following description of the operation sequence, these illustrations are shown in diminished size in every single operative step.

The core of the Operation Primer is the chapter **Nodal points.** This is where the actual sequence of the operation is described in detail. However, prior to this detailed explanation, the term nodal point will be covered briefly. In the foreword and introduction mental training was mentioned as a form of training used successfully in top-class sports for decades, and this is where the term originates. In sports as in surgery, a nodal point is understood as one of those structural components of movement that are absolutely essential for performing the movement optimally. Nodal points have to be passed through in succession and are characterized by a reduction in the degrees of freedom of action.

In mental training they act as orientation points for methodically repeated and conscious imagination of the athletic movement or operation (cf. in detail Immenroth, Eberspächer & Hermann, 2008).

For every operation in the Operation Primer series, these nodal points were extracted in a prolonged process by the authors in collaboration with the editors. The nodal

I	Preparations for the operation
II	Creating the pneumoperitoneum – placing the optical trocar
III	Placing the working trocars
IV	Nodal points
V	Management of difficult situations, complications and mistakes
VI	Anatomical variations
	Appendix

3 possibilities for creating the pneumoperitoneum: the choice is up to the surgeon

Veress needle = greatest danger!

Continuous illustration of the trocar positions

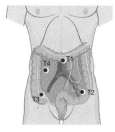

Nodal point = term from top-class sports

Nodal points:
1) absolutely essential
2) successive order
3) no degrees of freedom

Flow chart of the sequence of nodal points on each double page

points represent the basic structural framework of an operation. Because of their particular relevance and for better orientation, all of the nodal points in the Operation Primer are shown on the left on each double page as a flow chart. The current nodal point is highlighted graphically. The instruments required for this nodal point and the specific trocars for it are listed in a box on the right beside the flow chart.

Maximum of 7±2 instructions per nodal point

Below the instrument box, instructions regarding the nodal point are given as briefly as possible. Based on the ideas of Miller (1956), according to whom people can best store 7±2 information units ("Magical number 7"), not more than seven single instructions per nodal point are listed, if possible. With regard to the instructions, it should be noted that the change of instruments between the individual nodal points is not described explicitly as a rule; rather, this is apparent through different instruments in the instrument box.

Danger warnings are pointed out in red!

Where necessary, particular moments of danger are pointed out in red.

Alternatives: In small blue print at the end of the nodal point.

The described operation sequence is only one way of performing the operation safely and economically, namely the way preferred by the authors. Undoubtedly, a number of other equally valid operation sequences exist. As far as possible, notes on alternative methods are given in small blue print at the end of each nodal point.

In the fifth chapter, the **Management of difficult situations, complications and mistakes** is described in detail. In general, details on adhesions, bleeding, injuries to organs, etc. are given first.

Illustration of the most important anatomical variations

The following chapter goes into relevant **Anatomical variations** which can occur in the described operation sequence and may require a different approach. In order to provide a clear description, only the most important anatomical variations are mentioned.

Example of an operation note in the appendix

In order to give the Operation Primer even more practical relevance, an example of an operation note is reproduced in the **Appendix.** Besides the operation note, the appendix also contains the references and lists of key words.

(→ p. 61, V-4) = reference to the 4th section of chapter V

In order to avoid repetition, reference is made throughout the text to relevant chapters of the Operation Primer if necessary. To do this, the Roman numeral of the chapter and the number of the corresponding section are shown in brackets. Referral is made most often to the fifth chapter where the management of difficult situations, complications and mistakes is described. These references are set off in red letters.

All sources in the literature are listed in the bibliography

Additionally, it must be pointed out that for better readability of the Operation Primer no bibliographical references at all are given in the text. However, in order to give an overview of the basic and more extensive sources, the entire literature is listed in the bibliography.

Preparations for the operation

Make sure that the following preoperative requirements for laparoscopic sigmoidectomy have been met:

- the indication for the operation is correct,
- the patient has given detailed written consent,
- the bowel is prepared appropriately prior to laparoscopic colorectal surgery,
- thrombosis prophylaxis (low-molecular-weight heparin), and
- perioperative antibiotic prophylaxis (single shot) have been given.

- Size 11 scalpel
- 10-ml syringe and 0.9 % NaCl solution
- Dissecting scissors
- Langenbeck hooks
- Suction device
- Needle holder
- Suture scissors
- Forceps
- Backhaus clamps
- Compresses
- Swabs with an integral X-ray contrast strip

- Sutures:
  - Fascia: 2 – 0 absorbable, polyfilament
  - Subcutaneous: 3 – 0 absorbable, polyfilament
  - Skin: 2 – 0 or 3 – 0 non-absorbable, monofilament
  - Colon: 4 – 0 absorbable, monofilament

- Skin adhesive, if necessary
- Dressings

Instruments for the first access, depending on the type of access:

a) Hasson method
  - Hasson trocar (10/12 mm)
  - 2 retaining sutures (2 – 0)
  - Purse-string suture (2 – 0)

b) Trocar with optical obturator (e.g. Endopath XCEL® bladeless trocar, Ethicon Endo-Surgery)

c) Veress needle (e.g. Ultra Veress Needle, Ethicon Endo-Surgery)

> There should always be a basic laparotomy set in the operating room so that in an emergency a laparotomy can be performed without delay!

Additional laparoscopic instruments for sigmoidectomy

Trocars: (e.g. Endopath XCEL® trocar, Ethicon Endo-Surgery)

T1: Optical trocar   (10/12 mm)
T2: Working trocar   (5 mm or 10/12 mm)
T3: Working trocar   (10/12 mm)
T4: Working trocar   (5 mm or 10/12 mm)

* Additional trocars, if necessary
* Reducer caps, if necessary

* Angled optic (0° optic, if necessary for trocar with optical obturator)

Dissecting instruments:

* 2 atraumatic grasping forceps (5 mm and/or 10 mm)
* Curved dissector
* Ultrasonic dissector (e.g. Harmonic® shears or Harmonic ACE® shears, Ethicon Endo-Surgery)

> Before using Harmonic® instruments read the instructions for use and become familiar with the instrument!

* HF (high frequency) cautery electrode handle and forceps (for hemostasis in the subcutaneous fatty tissue)
* Curved scissors (for adhesions)

* Dissecting swab
* Suction-irrigation instrument
* Angulated retractor
* Endoscopic linear cutter (e.g. Endopath® ETS or Echelon 60® linear cutter, Ethicon Endo-Surgery)
* Additional cartridges, if necessary
* Transluminal circular stapler (e.g. Proximate® ILS circular stapler, Ethicon Endo-Surgery)
* Purse-string suture clamp (e.g. EH 40, Ethicon)
* Clip applier (e.g. Ligamax® or Absolok® clip applier, Ethicon Endo-Surgery/ Ethicon)
* Titanium or absorbable clips
* 3 Allis clamps
* Antiseptic solution
* Penrose drain

> Alternative: Instead of Harmonic® shears, bipolar scissors can be used for dissecting.

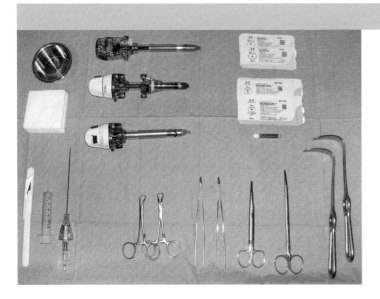

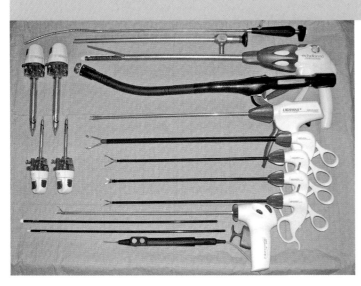

Emptying the bladder

- In order to avoid injuries to the bladder, make sure that the patient's bladder is emptied preoperatively by placing a temporary transurethral catheter.

Positioning of the patient

- Position the patient in the lithotomy position.
- Then tilt the table in an anti-Trendelenburg (10–20°) and right-lateral position (10°).
- Place the buttocks at the distal edge of the table and stretch thighs and legs apart with a slight flexure.
- Place the right arm alongside the body and the left arm at an angle no greater than 70° to the long axis of the body in order to avoid injuries to the axillary nerve.
- Use shoulder supports (both sides) and right lateral support or a vacuum mattress to prevent the patient from sliding when put in extreme positions.

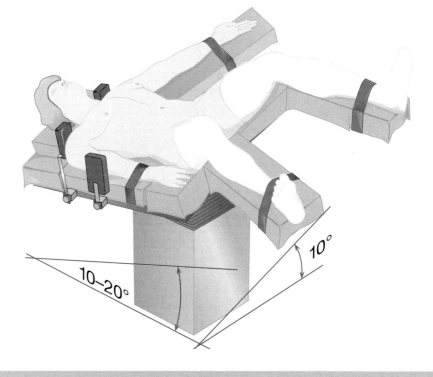

Shaving

- Shave the patient from the mamillae to above the pubic symphysis and from left to the right anterior superior iliac spine in order to be able to convert to a conventional operation if complications occur.
- If monopolar current is used, shave the adhesion side for the neutral electrode (as close as possible to the operating field, e.g. on the upper thigh).

- Before placing the neutral electrode, ensure that the skin at this site and all skin areas in contact with the table are absolutely dry.

- Then stick the entire surface of the electrode carefully above the greatest possible muscle mass. The conducting cable must be at the greatest possible distance from the operating field.

> When using monopolar current, always guard against burns on moist areas of the skin due to current!

Setting the equipment

- Set the generator of the HF or ultrasound dissector to an appropriate power level for the intended use.

- Position the foot pedal.

- Attach the suction-irrigation unit.

- Select a pressure plateau of maximally 12 mmHg on the CO_2 insufflator (with a flow of 6–8 l/min).

Skin disinfection

- Disinfect the skin from the mamillae to the pubic symphysis. Pay particular attention to careful disinfection of all skin folds.

Sterile draping

- Drape the operating field with sterile drapes so that it is limited cranially at the level of the xiphoid, just above the symphysis caudally and by the axillary lines laterally.

Positioning of the operating team

Lithotomy position

- The surgeon stands to the right at the level of the patient's abdomen.

- The camera assistant stands to the right at the level of the patient's head.

- The second assistant stands to the left at the level of the patient's abdomen.

- The instrument nurse stands to the right at the level of the patient's leg.

- One monitor is located in the line of vision of the surgeon and the camera assistant at the level of the patient's left leg.

- Another monitor is located in the line of vision of the second assistant on the right at the level of the patient's head.

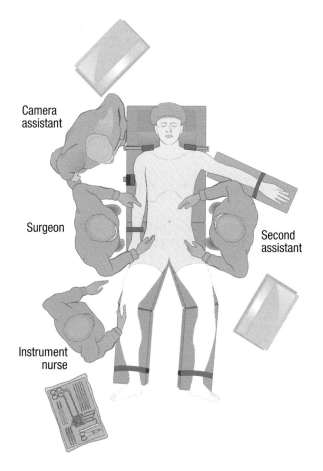

Camera assistant

Surgeon

Second assistant

Instrument nurse

Alternative: There is the possibility to operate without a second assistant. In that case the camera assistant stands to the left at the level of the patient's abdomen or, if convenient, to the right at the level of the patient's head.

Creating the pneumoperitoneum – placing the optical trocar

There are three ways of creating a pneumoperitoneum, which will be described in detail below:

a) Hasson method (open technique)

b) Trocar with optical obturator

c) Veress needle (closed technique)

Because of the large variety of trocars available and the resulting variety of methods of introducing the trocars, follow their individual instruction manuals!

a) Hasson method (open technique)

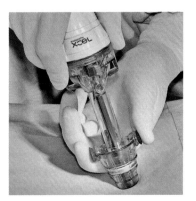

> Size 11 scalpel
>
> Scissors
>
> Forceps
>
> Langenbeck hook
>
> 2 retaining sutures (2–0)
>
> Purse-string suture (2–0)
>
> Hasson trocar (10/12 mm)

Incise the skin 2–3 cm above the umbilicus, making a 1.5- to 2-cm skin incision.

> **Ensure that the skin incision is the correct length:**
> - An incision that is too small can make insertion of the trocars much more difficult. If the skin around the trocars then suffers increased tension, this may later lead to skin necrosis!
> - An incision that is too large can result in gas loss and trocar dislocation (→ p. 61, V-4b)!

Spread the subcutaneous fat with the scissors as far as the linea alba. Try to stay midway between the two bellies of the rectus abdominis muscle. Use two Langenbeck hooks to expose the fascia of the anterior rectus sheath.

Then insert two 2–0 retaining sutures at the junction between the linea alba and the rectus muscle and draw the fascia upwards by pulling the sutures.

Use a scalpel to open the fascia between the two retaining sutures over a distance of 1.5 cm.

To expose the peritoneum, retract the fascia by repositioning the Langenbeck hooks.

Now lift the peritoneum with the forceps and incise it with the scissors over a length of about 1–1.5 cm. Check for the presence of close adhesions by inserting a finger into the incision site and palpating over the entire 360° circumference of the site.

Place a purse-string suture around the peritoneal incision and introduce the blunt Hasson trocar through the incision into the free abdominal cavity.

Secure the trocar with the two previously placed retaining sutures by tying them around the wings of the trocar cone. Tighten the purse-string suture around the Hasson trocar.

Secure the CO_2 supply tube to the trocar, remove the obturator and insufflate the gas until the preselected pressure of maximally 12 mmHg is reached.

> Alternative: There is a possibility to perform an open technique without the use of a Hasson trocar. After the incision of the peritoneum place a blunt stick through the incision in the free abdominal cavity, using it as a support for the placement of the optical trocar under vision control.

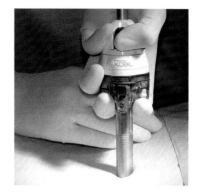

Size 11 scalpel

Trocar with optical obturator

Optic (0°)

Incise the skin 2–3 cm above the umbilicus, making a 1.5-cm skin incision.

> Ensure that the skin incision is the correct length:
> • An incision that is too small can make insertion of the trocars much more difficult. If the skin around the trocars then suffers increased tension, this may later lead to skin necrosis!
> • An incision that is too large can result in gas loss and trocar dislocation (→ p. 61, V-4b)!

Insert the optic into the optical obturator located in the trocar and lock it.

Place the transparent conical tip into the incision. Now carefully push the different layers of the abdominal wall tangentially apart by applying light pressure and using to-and-fro rotating movements of the blunt obturator tip. The special construction of the obturator allows the layers to be identified before they are pushed apart.

Perform this tissue separation and the final perforation of the peritoneum under constant vision.

> When bringing in the trocars, take care
> • to go in vertically,
> • to support the trocar with the hand, and
> • not to expend too much force in order to avoid organ injuries in case of resistance loss (→ p. 59, V-2; V-3)!

Finally, remove the optic together with the obturator from the trocar.

Secure the CO_2 supply tube to the trocar and insufflate the gas until the preselected pressure of maximally 12 mmHg is reached.

c) Veress needle (closed technique)

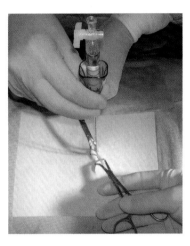

Inserting the Veress needle and the first trocar are the most dangerous moments in minimally invasive surgery, as the insertion is done "blind". There are many reported cases of major injuries to the aorta and the iliac artery caused by the use of the Veress needle!

Size 11 scalpel

Veress needle

10-ml syringe with NaCl solution

Optical trocar T1 (10/12 mm)

2 Backhaus clamps

Patients who have undergone previous surgery carry a higher risk of having adhesions! In these patients or in case of hepatomegaly, the Veress needle should never be used!

To minimize the risk of injury that may be caused by the Veress needle, select access in the left upper abdomen subcostally in the midclavicular line.

Incise the skin, making a 1.5- to 2-cm skin incision.

Elevate with the help of the assistant the abdominal wall with two Backhaus clamps, and carefully insert the Veress needle vertically with your hand supported above the skin incision. The penetration of the abdominal wall layers by the Veress needle can be felt or even heard.

When bringing in the Veress needle, take care
- to go in vertically (→ p. 61, V-4a),
- to support the hand holding the needle, and
- not to expend too much force in order to avoid organ injuries in case of loss of resistance (→ p. 59, V-2; V-3)!

Check the correct position of the Veress needle by applying the following obligatory safety tests:

Aspiration test
Attach a 10-ml syringe filled with NaCl solution to the Veress needle. It should be possible to aspirate air as a sign that the intra-abdominal position is correct.

Injection test
Inject NaCl solution through the Veress needle into the abdominal cavity. This can be done easily if it is in the correct position. Increased resistance of the syringe plunger indicates a possible incorrect position of the Veress needle.

Rotation test

Carefully rotate the slightly tilted needle inside the abdominal cavity. If the needle can be rotated freely, adhesions in the close vicinity are unlikely.

Slurp test

Apply one drop of NaCl solution onto the cone of the Veress needle, placing it convex on the opening. Now pull up the abdominal wall, making sure not to fix the Veress needle with your hand. Elevating the abdominal wall will create a partial vacuum, which in turn will cause the drop of NaCl to be sucked into the abdominal cavity, provided the Veress needle is correctly placed. A substantial vacuum will cause an additional "slurping" sound to be heard at the cone of the Veress needle.

If the safety tests indicate that the Veress needle has been placed correctly, attach the gas supply tube.

Excessively high intra-abdominal resting pressure and no flow indicate that the tip of the Veress needle is obstructed, e.g. by the greater omentum (→ **p. 59, V-3a**). In this case, perform the following test:

Manometer test

In order to release the Veress needle, manually lift up the abdominal wall. This should result in an obvious pressure drop. If this is not the case, remove the Veress needle and then place it again.

Insufflate the CO_2 until the preselected pressure of maximally 12 mmHg is reached (recommended maximum flow through the Veress needle: ~1.8 l/min). After that, remove the Veress needle from the skin incision.

To be sure that the Veress needle has been placed correctly, check for an adequate flow during the CO_2 insufflation and an appropriate increase in pressure on the insufflator!

Now place the optical trocar in the subumbilical skin incision. To do so use either

- a trocar with a sharp tip (10/12 mm) or
- a trocar with optical obturator.

When bringing in the trocars, take care
- to go in vertically,
- to support the trocar with the hand, and
- not to expend too much force in order to avoid organ injuries in case of loss of resistance (→ p. 59, V-2; V-3)!

Placing the working trocars

Optical trocar T1	(10/12 mm)
Working trocar T2	(5 mm or 10/12 mm)
Working trocar T3	(10/12 mm)
Working trocar T4	(5 mm or 10/12 mm)
Size 11 scalpel	
Reducer caps, if necessary	

Insert the optic into the trocar (T1).

In a diagnostic overview make sure that there are no pathological changes and/or injuries which might change the operative strategy or even prevent continuation of the operation (→ **p. 59, V-2; V-3**).

Choose the working trocar sites T2, T3, and T4 by palpating the abdominal wall under vision and use diaphanoscopy to ensure that no major cutaneous vessels will be injured when the trocars are inserted (→ **p. 59, V-1; V-2**).

> **T2:** In the left fossa iliaca
> **T3:** In the right fossa iliaca
> **T4:** In the right upper abdomen quadrant

Incise the skin with a scalpel according to the trocar diameter: about 1 cm when using a 5-mm trocar and 1.5 cm with a 10/12-mm trocar. Now insert the working trocars under vision.

Ensure that the skin incision is the right size!

When placing the trocars – particularly T3 and T4 – make sure they point exactly towards the operating field, as later corrections will not be possible.

When placing the trocars take care
- to insert the trocar under vision to avoid injuries (→ p. 59, V-2; V-3);
- to point the trocars exactly towards to the operation field, as later corrections will be difficult, if not impossible;
- to place additional trocars at any time to gain optimal conditions of work;
- to place the trocars with a minimum distance of 10 cm in order to avoid interference of camera and instruments;
- to pay attention to the distance between the trocars and the iliac spine (at least 1 cm distance)!

Remove the obturators from the trocars and attach the reducer caps to T2, T3 and T4, if necessary.

There are many ways to position the trocars.
We prefer the following way, but it should be the surgeon's choice!

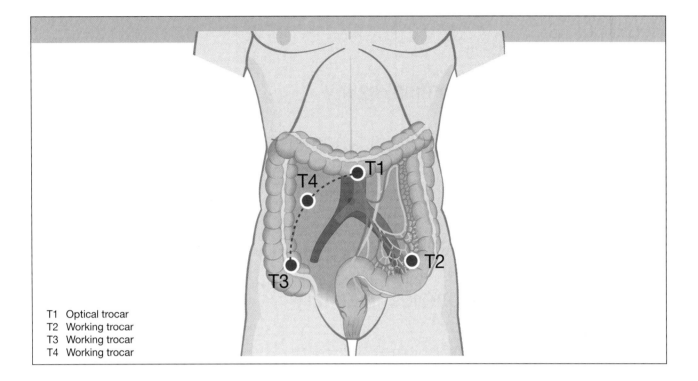

T1 Optical trocar
T2 Working trocar
T3 Working trocar
T4 Working trocar

Nodal points

1 Exploring the abdominal cavity

2 Identifying the anatomical landmarks

3 Mobilizing the left lateral colon

4 Mobilizing the splenic flexure

5 Dissecting the sigmoid mesentery

6 Dissecting the upper mesorectum

7 Dividing the upper rectum

8 Extracting the sigmoid

9 Dividing the proximal colon and preparing the anastomosis extra-abdominally

10 Preparing the anastomosis intra-abdominally

11 Anastomosing the colon

12 Verifying the anastomosis

13 Finishing the operation

Overview nodal points

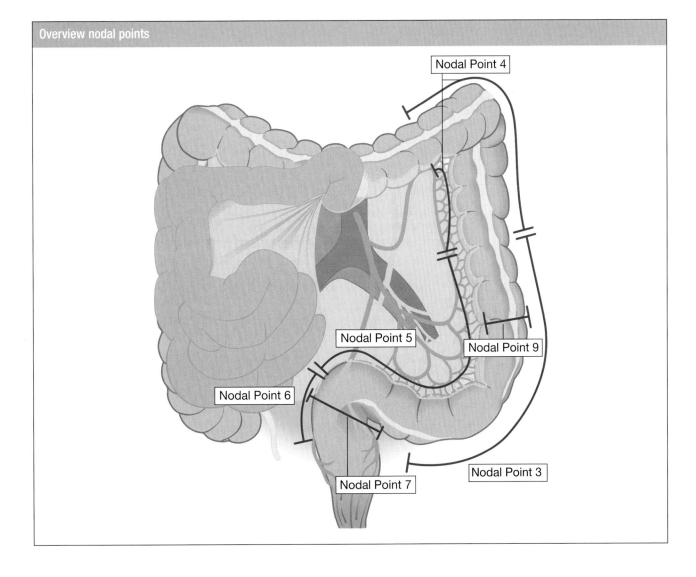

Nodal Point 4

Nodal Point 5

Nodal Point 9

Nodal Point 6

Nodal Point 7

Nodal Point 3

Nodal point 1　　　　　**Exploring the abdominal cavity**

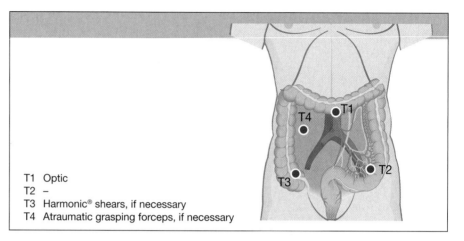

T1　Optic
T2　–
T3　Harmonic® shears, if necessary
T4　Atraumatic grasping forceps, if necessary

Examine the abdominal cavity carefully by inspecting it in a clockwise direction:

- Pelvis: dome of the bladder, Douglas pouch, the internal hernial orifices, uterus and adnexa in women
- Cecum with appendix
- Ascending colon
- Right upper abdomen: liver and gallbladder, right colonic flexure
- Greater omentum
- Transverse colon
- Left upper abdomen: stomach and spleen, splenic flexure
- Descending colon
- Sigmoid colon
- Jejunum and ileum

Look particularly for adhesions, erythema, vascular injections, serous fluids, pus and tumors.

> If a tumor is found during operation, the operative strategy has to be modified (e.g. conversion may be considered)!

Particularly check the trocar incision site for adhesions and possible bleeding. Change the optic position, if necessary (→ p. 59, V-1; V-2).

Divide any adhesions in the operating field using sharp dissection (→ p. 59, V-1).

> Divide any adhesions with organs promptly in order to avoid injuries (→ p. 59, V-3)!

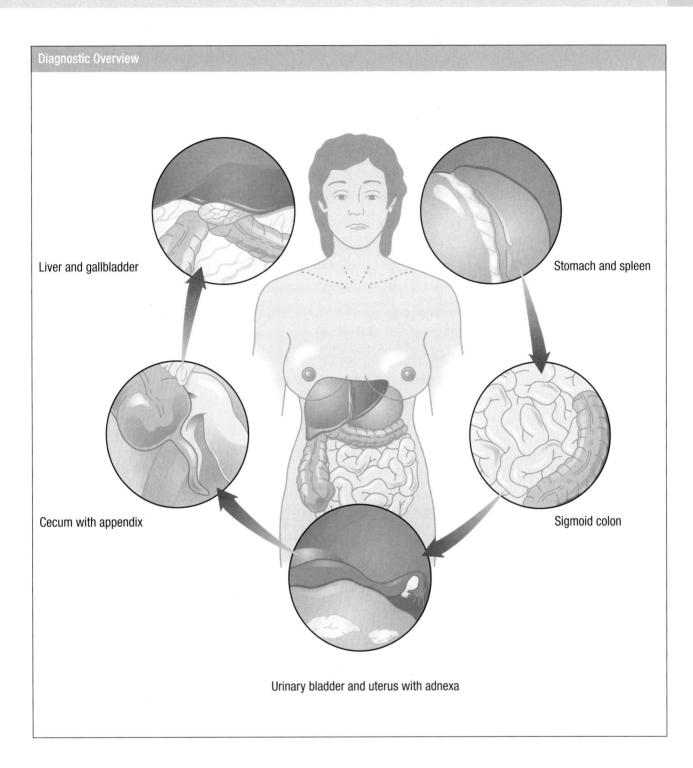

Liver and gallbladder

Stomach and spleen

Cecum with appendix

Sigmoid colon

Urinary bladder and uterus with adnexa

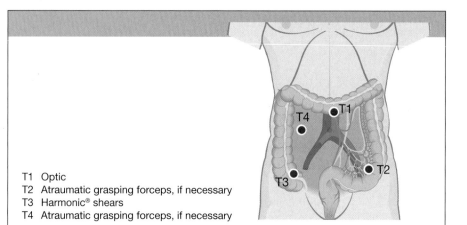

T1 Optic
T2 Atraumatic grasping forceps, if necessary
T3 Harmonic® shears
T4 Atraumatic grasping forceps, if necessary

Identify the following anatomical landmarks:

Lower abdomen:
- Sigmoid colon/sigmoid loop
- Rectum and rectosigmoid junction
- Inferior mesenteric artery
- Genital organs in women (uterus, adnexes)

Upper abdomen:
- Spleen
- Splenic flexure
- Transverse colon

Retract the jejunum to the right hypochondrium below the right transverse colon.

Place the distal portion of the small intestine in the right iliac fossa along with the cecum.

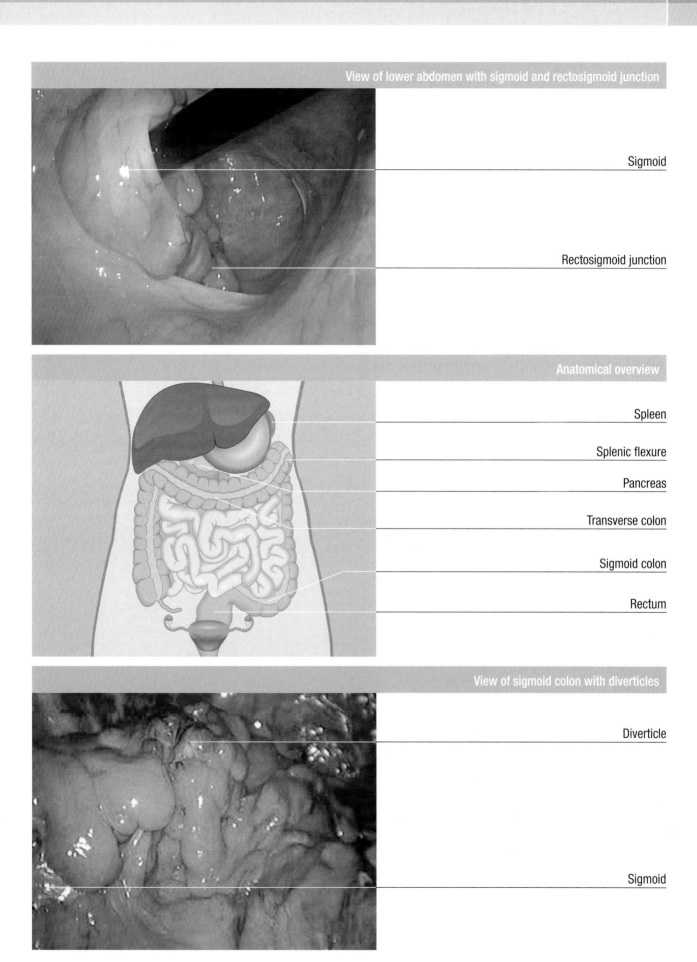

Sigmoid

Rectosigmoid junction

Anatomical overview

Spleen

Splenic flexure

Pancreas

Transverse colon

Sigmoid colon

Rectum

View of sigmoid colon with diverticles

Diverticle

Sigmoid

Nodal point 3   Mobilizing the left lateral colon

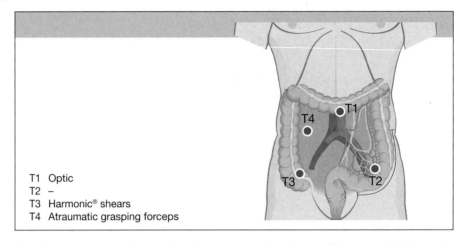

T1 Optic
T2 –
T3 Harmonic® shears
T4 Atraumatic grasping forceps

Put the patient in a right position in order to make the small intestine slide into the right abdomen by gravity (→ p. 20, I).

Dissect left lateral embryonic physiologic adhesions between peritoneum and the sigmoid colon with Harmonic® shears (T3) (→ p. 61, V-6).

Use a grasper through T4 to push the sigmoid loop medially.

Dissect in direction of the splenic flexure on the plane of Gerota's fascia.

In case of extensive lateral adhesions due to inflammation, perform a medial-posterior approach to avoid ureter damage.

> To avoid injuries to the ureter and iliac vessels identify them clearly. This can be difficult in case of inflammatory adhesions of the sigmoid to the abdominal wall (→ p. 61, V-6; V-7; p. 62, V-8)!

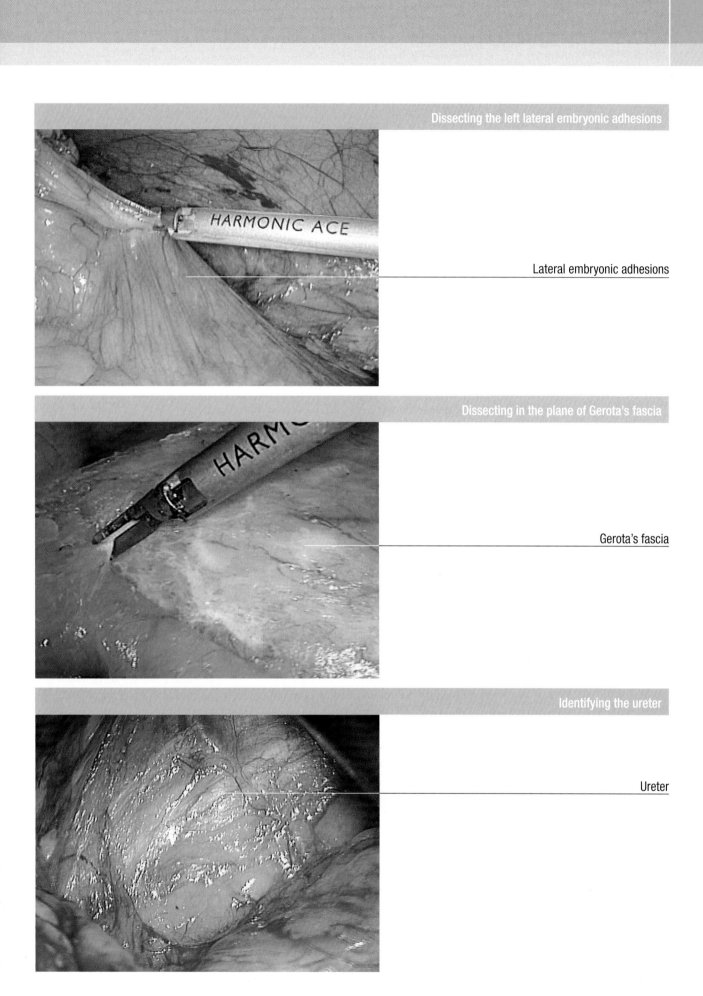

Dissecting the left lateral embryonic adhesions

Lateral embryonic adhesions

Dissecting in the plane of Gerota's fascia

Gerota's fascia

Identifying the ureter

Ureter

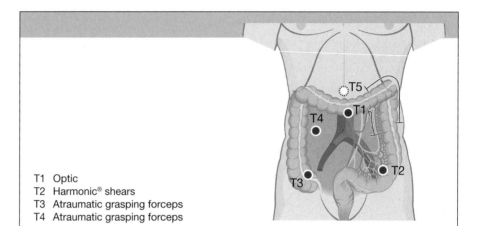

T1 Optic
T2 Harmonic® shears
T3 Atraumatic grasping forceps
T4 Atraumatic grasping forceps

To assure a tension-free anastomosis, dissect the splenic flexure and the left third of the transverse colon.

Put the patient in an anti-Trendelenburg position to reach the dissection area of the splenic flexure (→ p. 20, I). Dissect with Harmonic® shears (T2) the adhesions of the greater omentum and the splenocolic ligament in an anti-clockwise direction (→ p. 59, V-1).

Use the atraumatic grasper (T4) to smoothly tear the splenic flexure in a mediocaudal direction.

Mobilize the transverse colon till the inferior border of the pancreas while preserving the vascular supply of the transverse and proximal left colon.

Dissect the area of the transverse mesocolon carefully, as the inferior border of the pancreas has adhesions to the transverse mesocolon which can result in injuries of the pancreatic tail. It is sometimes difficult to distinguish the pancreatic tail from omental fat.

> Identify the pancreatic tail in order to avoid injuries of the pancreas
> (→ p. 60, V-3f)!

Loosen the adhesions of the greater omentum to the colon while staying close to the colon (→ p. 59, V-1).

> Alternative: If the patient has a high splenic flexure introduce an additional trocar
> (T5) above T1 in the medial abdominal line. Introduce an atraumatic grasper in
> T5 and keep the greater omentum away. Change Harmonic® shears to T4 and
> dissect the splenic flexure from this position.

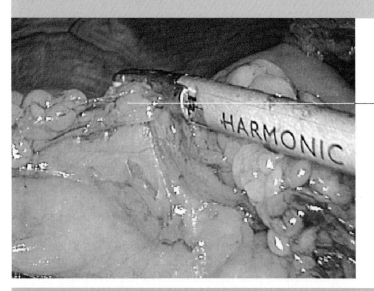

Spleen

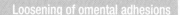

Omental fat

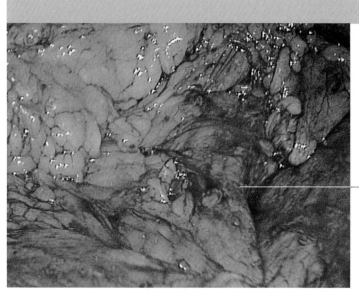

Lower margin of pancreatic tail

Nodal point 5   **Dissecting the sigmoid mesentery**

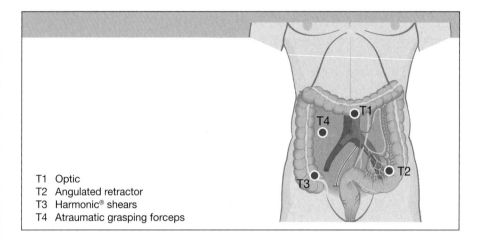

T1   Optic
T2   Angulated retractor
T3   Harmonic® shears
T4   Atraumatic grasping forceps

Put the patient into Trendelenburg position.

Incise and fenestrate the peritoneum of the sigmoid mesentery with Harmonic® shears (T3) and insert the angulated retractor (T2). Use the retractor to achieve an excellent exposure of the mesentery by elevating the sigmoid to the abdominal wall.

Dissect in the anatomic plane below the inferior mesenteric artery and the superior rectal artery and continue opening the mesentery aboral. During preparation reposition the angulated retractor to maintain continuous tension on the meso-sigmoid, and stay close to the colon in order to avoid injury to the left colic artery, the trunk of the sigmoid artery and the superior rectal artery.

> Preserve the left colic artery, the trunk of the sigmoid artery and the superior rectal artery, as in benign disease excellent blood circulation of the rectum is assured through preservation of the inferior mesenteric artery and the superior rectal artery (→ p. 59, V-2)!

Marginal arteries in the mesentery can be dissected with Harmonic® shears.

Identify the ureter, the hypogastric nerve structure and the genital blood vessels that cross the iliac vessels running into the pelvis. Dissect the avascular space in between Toldt's fascia and the mesentery for posterior and lateral freeing of the sigmoid.

> Make sure that the left ureter is clearly identified before posterior and lateral freeing of the sigmoid, and pay attention to the hypogastric nerve structure, genital blood vessels and iliac vein in order to avoid injuring them (→ p. 59, V-2; p. 61, V-7; p. 62, V-8)!

Continue the dissection of the mesentery at Toldt's line, staying in the avascular plane until the entire "high pressure zone" (including the rectosigmoid junction) is prepared.

> Alternative: Clip and divide the marginal arteries in the mesentery.

Aorta

Inferior mesenteric artery

Dissection line

Sigmoid colon

Sigmoid arteries

Superior rectal artery

Exposing the sigmoid mesentery for dissection

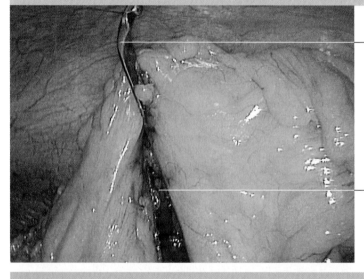

Angulated retractor

Fenestrated mesosigmoid

Dissecting the sigmoid mesentery with marginal sigmoid artery

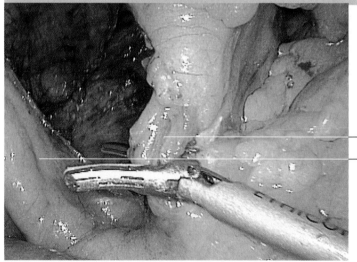

Marginal sigmoid artery

Mesosigmoid

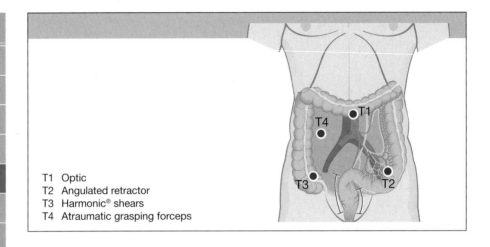

T1 Optic
T2 Angulated retractor
T3 Harmonic® shears
T4 Atraumatic grasping forceps

Determine the lower margin of resection in the upper rectum, which should be located in non-inflamed tissue (→ p. 62, V-10).

Use the loss of the appendices epiploicae and taeniae coli and the first collateral branch of superior rectal vessels as a landmark for the rectosigmoid junction.

> Don't use the position of the peritoneal fold of Douglas as a landmark, as there are numerous anatomical variations!

Dissect the mesorectum posteriorly with Harmonic® shears (T3), then laterally, until a sufficient distal margin is achieved. The mesorectum on the left side is closely attached to the parietal fascia where the superior hypogastric nerve and the left ureter are located; therefore, dissect carefully the left lateral side to avoid an anastomic leakage.

> Dissect the left lateral side of the mesorectum carefully to avoid injuries to the superior hypogastric nerve and the left ureter (→ p. 61, V-7)!

Dissect the first superior rectal artery and vein.

Clean the rectal wall while avoiding thermal damage (→ p. 60, V-3b).

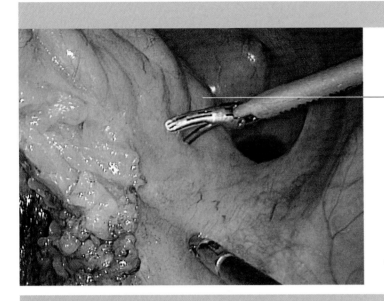

Mesorectum

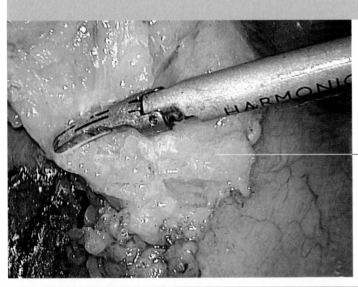

Mesorectum

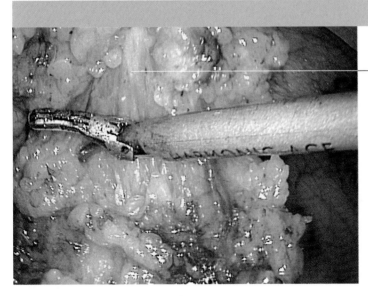

Rectal wall

Nodal point 7   **Dividing the upper rectum**

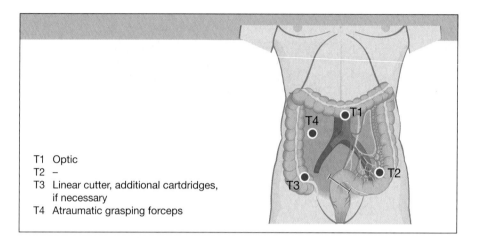

T1 Optic
T2 –
T3 Linear cutter, additional cartridges, if necessary
T4 Atraumatic grasping forceps

Before dividing the upper rectum, perform a transanal washout.

Open the jaws of the linear cutter and place them around the rectum at the level of the determined division line perpendicular to the digestive tract.

Close the linear cutter. In case of difficulties in closing the cutter, reposition the jaws and grasp less tissue. An accumulation of tissue at the proximal end of the jaws may result in an incomplete staple line.

> Make sure that there is no accumulated tissue at the proximal end of the jaws of the linear cutter to avoid an insufficient staple line that may lead to anastomotic leakage (→ p. 62, V-10)!

Fire the linear cutter.

Open the jaws of the linear cutter and make sure tissue is cleared from the jaws. Then close the jaws and remove the linear cutter.

In case of a large diameter of the rectum, place and fire the linear cutter again with additional cartridges until the rectum is totally divided.

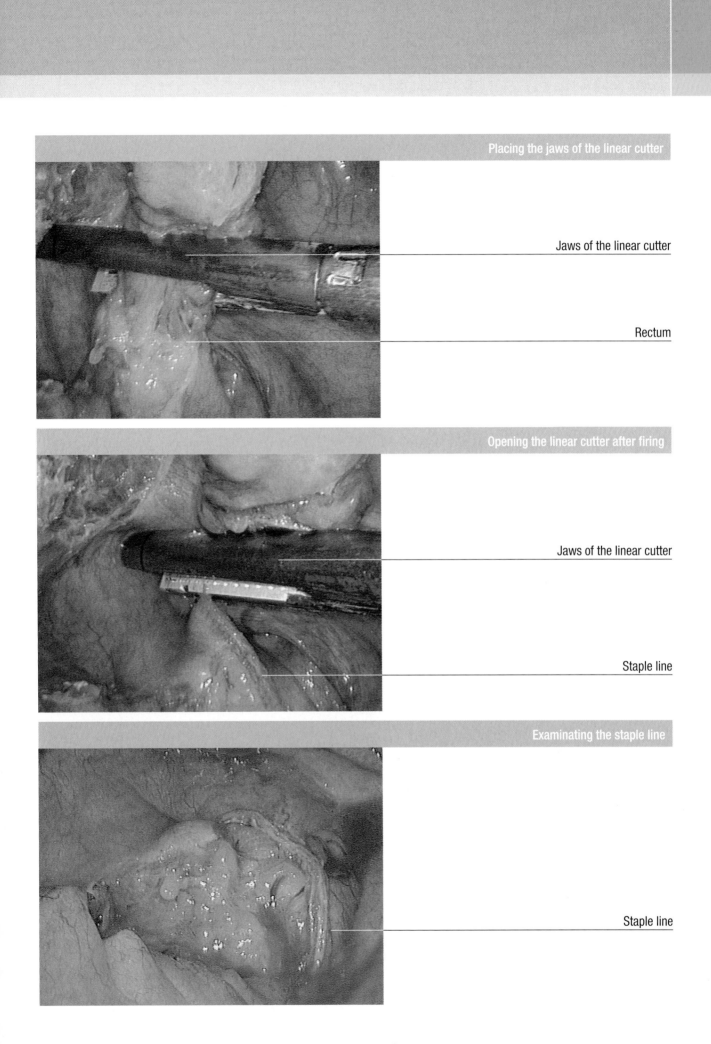

Placing the jaws of the linear cutter

Jaws of the linear cutter

Rectum

Opening the linear cutter after firing

Jaws of the linear cutter

Staple line

Examinating the staple line

Staple line

T1 Optic
T2 Atraumatic grasping forceps
T3 –
T4 –

Scalpel
Retractors

Widen the left lower incision of T2 to 4 cm length for extraction of the resected sigmoid. The incision size depends on the volume of specimen, patient's habitus, and cosmetic concerns.

Grasp the cut end of the resected sigmoid with an atraumatic grasping forceps (T2).

Remove trocar T2 while pulling out the resected sigmoid with the atraumatic grasping forceps. Widen the incision with retractors.

Alternative: Perform an incision in the suprapubic region (Pfannenstiel incision) for extraction of the resected sigmoid.

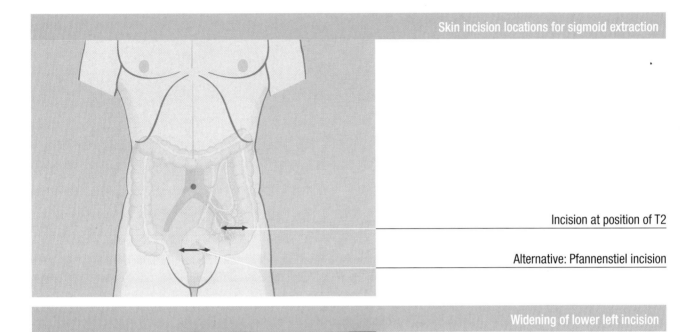

Incision at position of T2

Alternative: Pfannenstiel incision

Widening of lower left incision

Trocar T2

Extracting the sigmoid colon

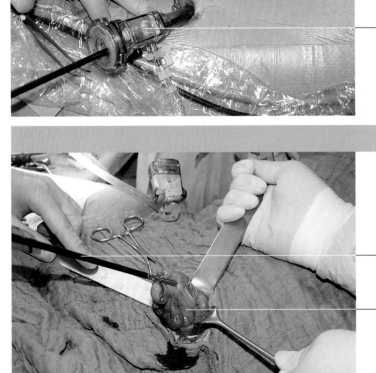

Atraumatic grasping forceps

Cut end of sigmoid

Nodal point 9   **Dividing the proximal colon and preparing the anastomosis extra-abdominally**

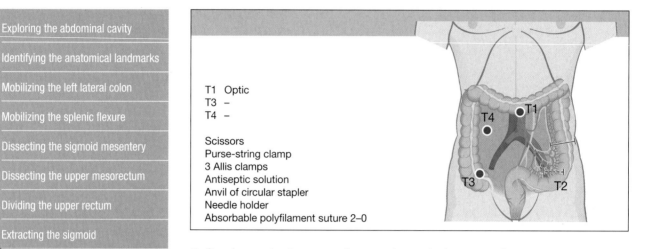

T1 Optic
T3 –
T4 –

Scissors
Purse-string clamp
3 Allis clamps
Antiseptic solution
Anvil of circular stapler
Needle holder
Absorbable polyfilament suture 2–0

Define the proximal resection line in a diverticle-free non-inflamed zone. Check for a proper blood supply by transecting the mesosigmoidal vessel (drummond's arcade).

Position a purse-string clamp, make a purse-string suture and dissect the specimen with scissors. Then place three Allis clamps and clean the lumen of the colon with an antiseptic solution.

Introduce the anvil (at least 29 mm in diameter) into the colonic lumen and close the purse-string suture.

Replace the prepared colon into the lower abdominal cavity and close the abdominal layers by primary closure with an absorbable polyfilament suture. Perform an intra-cutaneous wound closure.

Alternative: Make a hand-sewn purse-string suture.

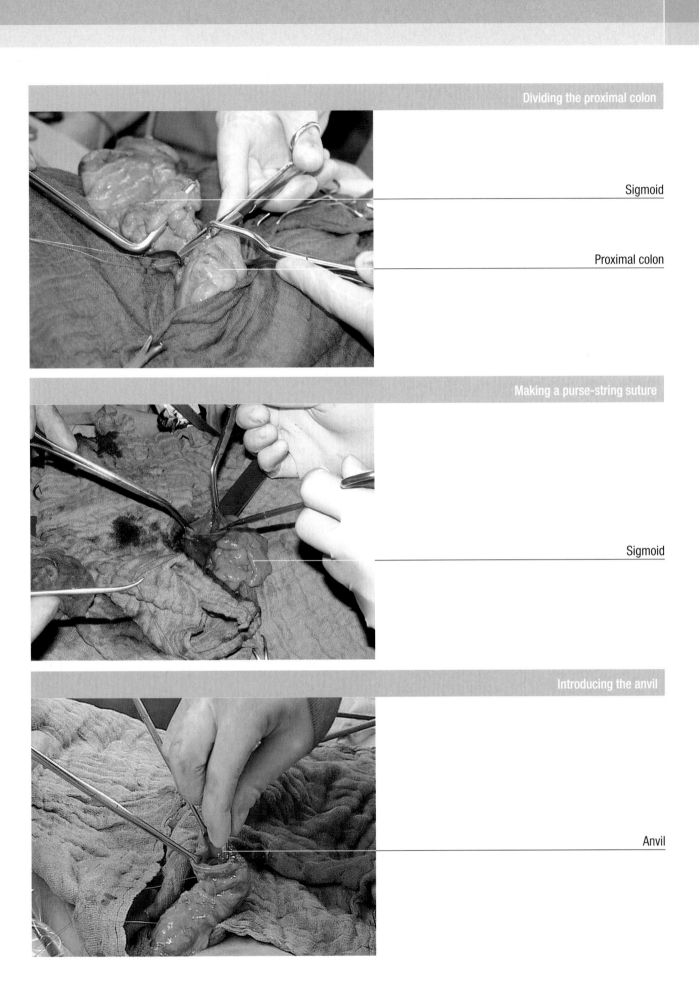

Sigmoid

Proximal colon

Sigmoid

Anvil

Nodal point 10   **Preparing the anastomosis intra-abdominally**

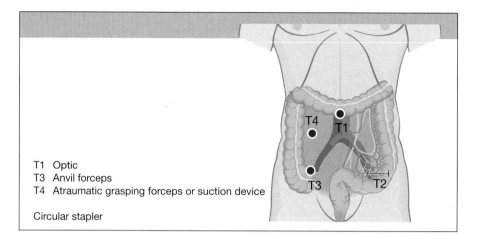

T1 Optic
T3 Anvil forceps
T4 Atraumatic grasping forceps or suction device

Circular stapler

Reestablish the pneumoperitoneum.

Before performing the anastomosis be aware that this is the most decisive step of the procedure and should be performed precisely.

> Be aware that any mistake could lead to serious complications subsequently (→ p. 62, V-10; V-11)!

First perform an atraumatic dilatation of the anus. Then introduce the circular stapler through the anus into the rectum.

Determine the perforation location for the trocar shaft, which is optimally placed directly above or below the staple line.

Afterwards perforate the rectal stump with the trocar shaft of the circular stapler. Turn the instrument gently while holding the knob. Use the anvil forceps (T3) to facilitate the perforation of the rectal stump.

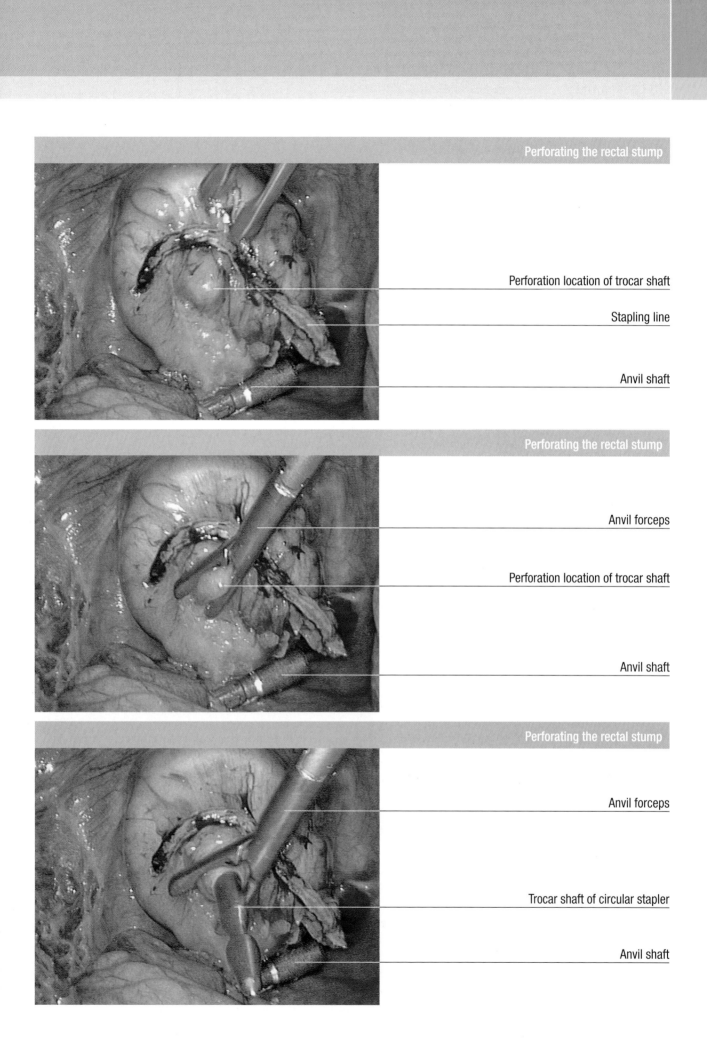

Perforation location of trocar shaft

Stapling line

Anvil shaft

Anvil forceps

Perforation location of trocar shaft

Anvil shaft

Anvil forceps

Trocar shaft of circular stapler

Anvil shaft

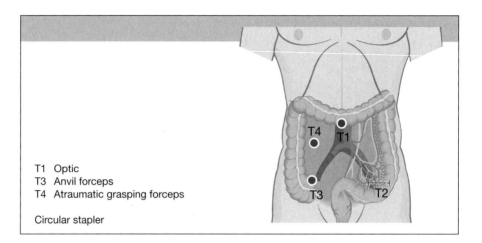

T1   Optic
T3   Anvil forceps
T4   Atraumatic grasping forceps

Circular stapler

Use the anvil forceps (T3) to connect the anvil shaft to the trocar shaft of the circular stapler.

With the optic (T1) inspect the descending colon up to the flexure and make sure that the proximal colon is not twisted.

> Before approximating colon and rectum make sure that the proximal colon is not twisted, to enable a tension-free anastomosis (→ p. 62, V-11)!

Pull back the circular stapler gently to prevent the appearance of anastomosis stenosis.

Close the circular stapler by turning the knob in a clockwise direction so that the colon and rectum will be approximated.

Before taking the next step, make sure that no neighboring organs are incarcerated (e.g. vagina, adnexa). In women, retract the posterior vaginal wall and perform a digital vaginal examination in case of doubt.

> Be aware that there is a high risk of incarcerating neighboring organs (e.g. vagina, adnexa) while doing the anastomosis!

Fire the device when appropriate in the gap-setting scale by squeezing the firing handle. A click should be heard, indicating a proper staple formation and cutting of tissue.

Open the circular stapler; rotate the knob anticlockwise by ½ to ¾.

> Notice that these instructions apply for the Proximate® ILS circular stapler (Ethicon Endo-Surgery). Before using another type of circular stapler read the instruction manual carefully!

Turn the instrument 90° on each side to make sure that the anvil is loosened completely from the surrounding tissue and withdraw it through the anus. Smoothly rotate the circular stapler while it is being extracted.

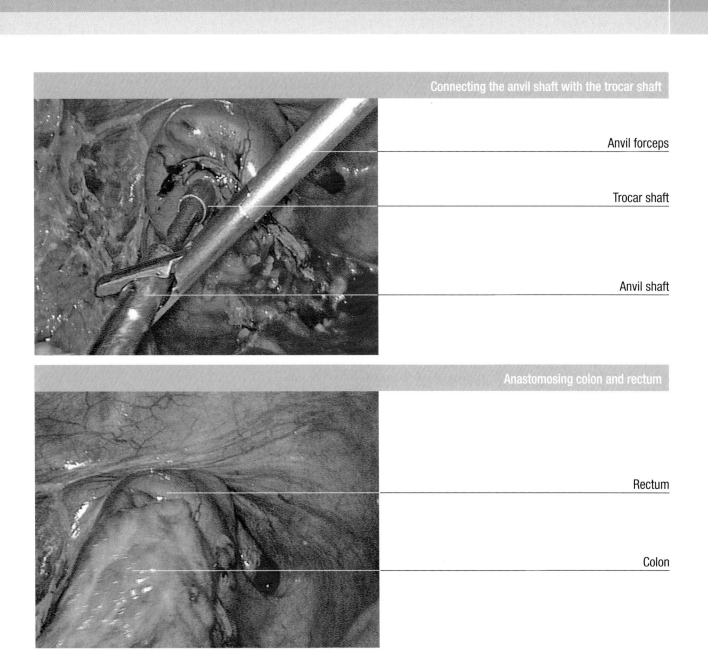

Connecting the anvil shaft with the trocar shaft

Anvil forceps

Trocar shaft

Anvil shaft

Anastomosing colon and rectum

Rectum

Colon

Nodal point 12   **Verifying the anastomosis**

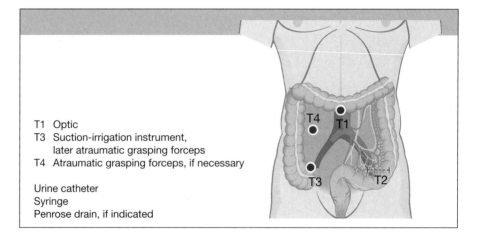

T1   Optic
T3   Suction-irrigation instrument,
      later atraumatic grasping forceps
T4   Atraumatic grasping forceps, if necessary

Urine catheter
Syringe
Penrose drain, if indicated

First check for circular aspects of the amputated rectal and colonic rings ("doughnuts"). Two complete "doughnuts" should be seen.

Then verify the anastomosis with an insufflation test. Fill the small pelvis with water using the suction-irrigation instrument (T3) and insufflate about 100 ml air, using a urine catheter connected to a syringe while the proximal colon is closed with an instrument. Look for bubbles, indicating an incomplete anastomosis (→ p. 62, V-10).

If in doubt, redo the insufflation test.

> It is mandatory to verify the completeness of the anastomosis before terminating the surgery (→ p. 62, V-10)!

Insert a Penrose drain in the small pelvis with an atraumatic grasping forceps (T3), if indicated.

> Alternative: Instead of an insufflation test an endoscopic transanal evaluation of the anastomosis can be performed.

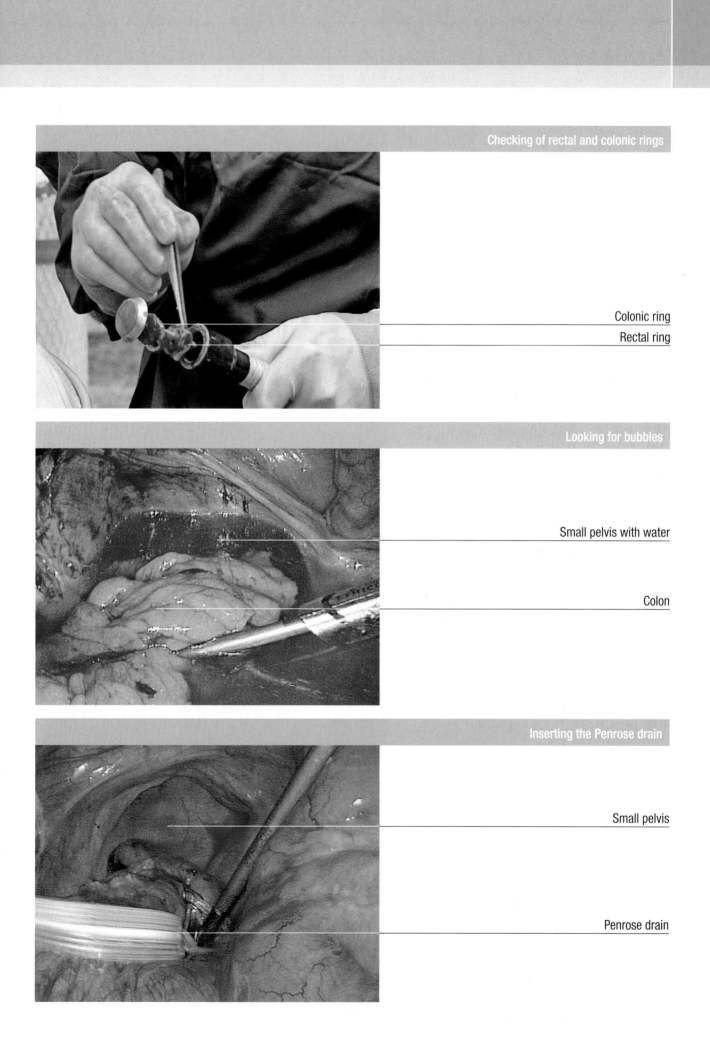

Colonic ring

Rectal ring

Small pelvis with water

Colon

Small pelvis

Penrose drain

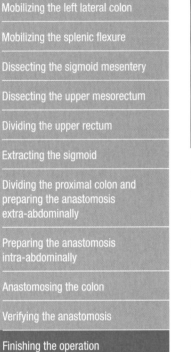

T1　Optic
T3　Penrose drain
T4　–

Fascia sutures: 2–0 absorbable, polyfilament
Subcutaneous sutures: 3–0 absorbable,
　polyfilament, if necessary
Skin sutures: 4–0 or 5–0 monofilament

Remove working trocars T3 and T4 carefully under vision to avoid a dislocation of the drain in T3.

Control the trocar incisions with regard to possible bleeding (→ p. 59, V-2).

Remove the optic and open the valve on the optical trocar for disinflation. Then remove the optical trocar.

Close the fascia where 10/12 mm trocars have been introduced.

Finally, close all incisions and cover the wounds with sterile dressings following disinfection.

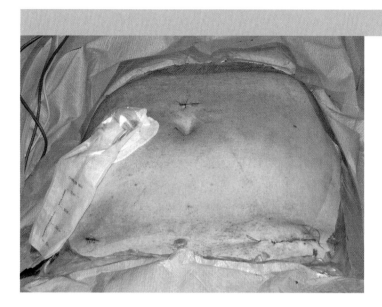

Management of difficult situations, complications and mistakes

In principle, the decision to proceed to laparotomy should be made too early rather than too late!
Convert immediately if the situation cannot be controlled laparoscopically!

Separate adhesions using Harmonic® shears or bipolar scissors as close to the abdominal wall as possible so as not to injure any organs.

a) Diffuse bleeding / bleeding from minor vessels

Coagulate the bleeding vessel with Harmonic® shears. If this does not terminate the bleeding, place a clip on the bleeding vessel.

b) Bleeding from major vessels

If large vessels such as the aorta, portal vein or vena cava are injured during the operation, open the abdomen immediately for vascular surgical treatment of the injury!

In case of injuries in which the extent cannot be determined with certainty, open the abdominal cavity for open management of the injury!

a) Greater omentum

Injury of the greater omentum can occur when the Veress needle is inserted too deeply and/or without elevation of the abdominal wall. All the safety tests may be positive so that the complication can be identified only when the optical trocar and the optic are inserted.

Manage any bleeding that occurs with Harmonic® shears. If, as a result of the insertion, the greater omentum is inflated like a tent, withdraw the optical trocar as far as the peritoneal margin and tap the abdomen with the flat hand. The omentum should then separate from the inside of the abdominal wall and collapse.

b) Bowel

Bowel injuries are the most frequent organ injuries in minimally invasive surgery. They are usually caused by instruments, especially by the Veress needle. Undissected adhesions can also be a cause of bowel injuries.

Manage bowel injuries by laparoscopic oversewing. If sufficient closure of the injury is not guaranteed, perform laparotomy. Irrigate the operating field gently with an antiseptic solution. As bowel resections always require a systemic antibiotic (single shot), the patient should already have antibiotic coverage.

c) Spleen

The splenic capsule is usually injured by traction when the colon is in close proximity to the spleen.

Reduction of splenic injury risk can be achieved by
- early (posterior) dissection of the splenocolic ligament before medialization of the splenic flexure and
- dissection of the flexure close to the colonic wall.

Bleeding from the spleen is ideally treated with Harmonic® shears. Alternatively, apply a hemostyptic. Laparotomy is the exception.

d) Stomach

If the gastric wall has been injured or perforated, oversew the affected area.

If necessary, perform an intra-operative gastroscopy.

e) Liver

Manage minor bleeding from the liver by brief compression with a swab, point contact with Harmonic® shears.

In the case of major hemorrhage which can be still controlled laparoscopically, apply a hemostyptic.

f) Pancreas

Manage minor bleeding from the pancreas by brief compression with a swab, point contact with Harmonic® shears.

In the case of major hemorrhage which can be still controlled laparoscopically, apply a hemostyptic.

To avoid pancreatic fistula it is recommended to insert a Penrose drain.

a) Veress needle

If the emphysema has occurred because of an incorrectly placed needle, remove the needle and reinsert it as described above (→ p. 26, II c). Ensure particularly that the angle of insertion is vertical and that the abdominal wall is lifted.

b) Trocar

Withdrawing a trocar so far that its opening comes to lie in front of the peritoneum is another cause of emphysema.

In this case, under vision push the trocar back into the correct position through the existing incision.

Losing a swab in the abdominal cavity 5

After losing a swab, fix the trocar in its last position and, under vision, look for the swab where it was lost, using grasping forceps.

Do not change the patient's position, and do not irrigate the abdominal cavity!

If necessary, search for the swab with the C-arm or perform a laparotomy to retrieve the swab.

Adhesion of the sigmoid to the abdominal wall 6

Inflammation of the sigmoid in diverticulitis often results in adhesions of the sigmoid to the abdominal wall. In this case, lateral mobilization can be difficult and there is a danger of injuring the ureter.

Use a medial posterior approach to identify the ureter in a healthy non-inflamed area.

Injury of the left ureter 7

With a medial approach, it can easily happen that the dissection is too deep and the left ureter is injured.

If the ureter is injured during mobilization or devascularization of the left colon, make a mini-incision in the left lateral abdomen immediately above the area of ureteral injury. The ureter may then be stented and repaired under direct vision. Following repair of the ureter, the mini-incision is used for specimen extraction, resection and completion of the anastomosis.

8 Injury of the iliac vessels

If the iliac vessels are injured during dissection of the mesosigmoid perform a laparoscopic compression of the vessels and make a mini-incision in the left lower abdomen immediately above the superficial to the iliac vessel injury. Repair the injured vessels under direct vision.

9 Difficulties when clipping

a) Incorrectly positioned clips

If an incorrectly positioned clip is the cause of bleeding from the inferior mesenteric artery, take care of the bleeding by compressing the vessel using grasping forceps, and then place a new clip at the correct point or tie up the vessel using an Endo ligature.

b) Unsafely positioned clips

If the lumen of the structure to be clipped is too big for complete closure, use a Roeder loop.

c) Lost and slipped clips

In case a previously placed clip has slipped, first of all replace it. Then find the slipped clip and remove it from the abdominal cavity.

10 Positive anastomotic leak test

If the leak test is positive, the anastomosis must be repaired or revised.

If the site of leakage is visible and is located on the anterior aspect of the colon, place laparoscopic sutures for repair and repeat the leak test.

If the site of leakage is difficult to identify, dissect and divide the rectum distal to the anastomosis and redo the anastomosis.

In cases where laparoscopic repair is not feasible, make a small laparotomy (either a Pfannenstiel incision or low midline incision) and redo the anastomosis by an open technique.

11 Rotation of the left colon

During laparoscopic sigmoidectomy, in rare cases, the proximal segment of the colon can be rotated when the specimen is being removed through a small incision. Rotation of the left colon will cause tension on the colonic anastomosis.

Therefore, it is advisable to inspect the position of the colon before the stapler is fired.

Anatomical variations

Short and straight sigmoid, obliquely protracted into the pelvis

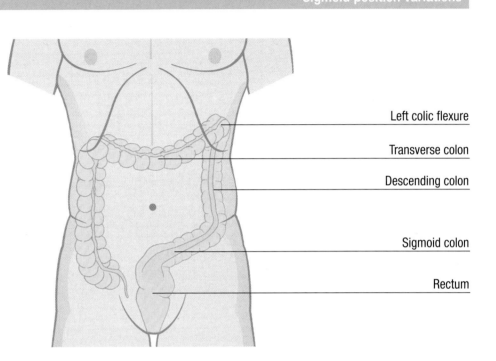

Left colic flexure

Transverse colon

Descending colon

Sigmoid colon

Rectum

The sigmoid colon forming a loop to the right

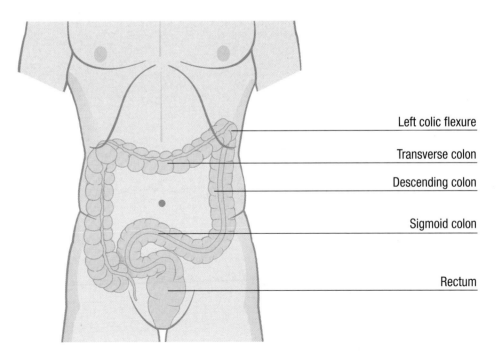

Left colic flexure

Transverse colon

Descending colon

Sigmoid colon

Rectum

Sigmoid position variations

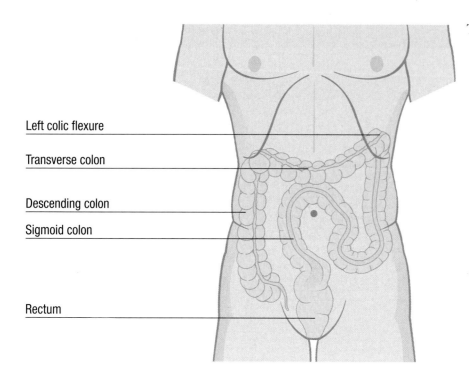

The sigmoid colon ascending highly

Left colic flexure

Transverse colon

Descending colon

Sigmoid colon

Rectum

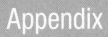
Sample operation note

Bibliography

List of key words

Sample operation note

Date:	Operating Surgeon:
Patient's name:	Assistant:
Operation diagnosis: Diverticulitis	Instrument nurse:
Operation: Laparoscopic sigmoidectomy	Anesthetist:

Patient under general anesthesia. Lithotomy position with adequate padding.

Following skin disinfection and sterile draping, introduction of 10/12 mm trocar in open technique in the median line, two fingers above the umbiculus. Introduction of optic, establishing of pneumoperitoneum and placing of two working trocars (10/12 mm) in the left and right lower abdomen and of a 5-mm trocar in the right middle abdomen.

Inspection of the abdominal cavity. Positioning of the patient to the right, using gravity to translocate small intestine. Start of colon preparation by detachment of left lateral embryonic adhesions to the abdominal wall. Identification of ureter and mobilization of left colon in the layer on the fascia of Gerota. In the area of the left colonic flexure dissection of the spleno-colic ligament and mobilization of the left part of the transverse colon.

Positioning of patient in Trendelenburg position. Fenestration of mesocolon on the transition of the colon descendens to the sigmoid. Dissection of mesocolon to the upper rectum. As landmarks for identifying the upper rectum the disappearing taenia libera, the promontorium and the appearance of geminated branches of the rectal arteries are used. Definition of distal division line.

Dissection of mesorectum with ultracision and posterior washout. Division of rectum between the upper and middle third with an linear cutter. Insufflation test of the staple line via the rectum.

Widening of the left lower trocar incision to a length of 3–4 cm and exteriorization of colon. Blood flow of the border of the vessel arcade is checked. Division of colon in the middle of the colon descendens. A purse-string suture is made and a 29-mm anvil is introduced. The colon with the anvil is replaced into the abdomen. Closing of the abdominal wall in layers.

Anastomosis of the colon descendens with the rectum is performed under vision. Colonic rings are checked for thickness and integrity. Transrectal air insufflation for verification of anastomosis.

Irrigation of operation field and positioning of a Penrose drain in the trocar of the right middle abdomen. Removal of trocars and checking for bleeding. Closing of fascia where 10/12-mm trocars have been used. Skin disinfection, skin sutures and dressings.

Ayoub S.F. (1978). Arterial supply to the human rectum. *Acta Anat,* 100: 317-327.

Carpenter W.B. (1874). *Principles of Mental Physiology: With their Applications to the Training and Discipline of the Mind and the Study of its Comorbid Conditions.* London: Henry S. King & Co.

Darzi A., Super P., Guillou P.J. & Monson J.R. (1994). Laparoscopic sigmoid colectomy: Total laparoscopic approach. *Dis Colon Rectum,* 37: 268-271.

Driskell J., Cooper C. & Moran A. (1994). Does mental practice enhance performance? *Journal of Applied Psychology,* 79: 481-492.

Eberspächer H. (2001). *Mentales Training.* München: Copress.

Feltz D.L. & Landers D.M. (1983). The effects of mental practice on motor skill learning and performance: A meta-analysis. *Journal of Sport Psychology,* 5: 25-57.

Fischer F. & Bruch H.P. (2006). Surgical principles in the treatment of diverticular disease. *Zentralbl Chir,* 131: W72-W81.

Geis W.P., Coletta A.V., Verdeja J.C., Plasencia G., Ojogho O. & Jacobs M. (1994). Sequential psychomotor skills development in laparoscopic colon surgery. *Arch Surg,* 129: 206-212.

Germer C.T., Ritz J.P. & Buhr H.J. (2003). Laparoskopische Kolonchirurgie. *Chirurg,* 4: 966-982.

Güler A.K., Immenroth M., Berg T., Bürger T. & Gawad K.A. (2006). Evaluation einer neu konzipierten Operationsfibel durch den Vergleich mit einer klassischen Operationslehre. *Posterpräsentation auf dem 123. Kongress der Deutschen Gesellschaft für Chirurgie vom 02.-05. Mai 2006 in Berlin.*

Immenroth M. (2003). *Mentales Training in der Medizin. Anwendung in der Chirurgie und Zahnmedizin.* Hamburg: Kovač.

Immenroth M., Bürger T., Brenner J., Kemmler R., Nagelschmidt R., Eberspächer H. & Troidl H. (2005). Mentales Training in der Chirurgie. *Der Chirurg BDC,* 44(1): 21-25.

Immenroth M., Bürger T., Brenner J., Nagelschmidt R., Eberspächer H. & Troidl H. (2007). Mental Training in surgical education: A randomized controlled trial. *Ann Surg,* 245: 385-391.

Immenroth M., Eberspächer H. & Hermann H.D. (2008). Training kognitiver Fertigkeiten. In J. Beckmann & M. Kellmann (Hrsg.), *Enzyklopädie der Psychologie (D, V, 2) Anwendungen der Sportpsychologie* (119-176). Göttingen: Hogrefe.

Bibliography

Immenroth M., Eberspächer H., Nagelschmidt M., Troidl H., Bürger T., Brenner J., Berg T., Müller M. & Kemmler R. (2005). Mentales Training in der Chirurgie – Sicherheit durch ein besseres Training. Design und erste Ergebnisse einer Studie. *MIC,* 14: 69-74.

Jung G. (1996). *Pflegestandards in der mininal-invasiven Chirurgie.* Hannover: Schlüterscher Verlag.

Köckerling F. (1995). Offene Laparoskopie. In Kremer K., Platzer W. & Schreiber H.W. (Hrsg.), *Chirurgische Operationslehre. Minimal-invasive Chirurgie, Band 7 Teil 2* (54-58). Stuttgart, New York: Georg Thieme Verlag.

Kwok S.P., Lau W.Y., Carey P.D., Kelly S.B., Leung K.L. & Li A.K. (1996). Prospective evaluation of laparoscopic-assisted large bowel excision for cancer. *Ann Surg,* 223: 170-176.

Lacy A.M., Garcia-Valdecasas J.C., Delgado S., Sabater L., Grande L., Fuster J. & Visa J. (1998). Unusual intraoperative complication in laparoscopic sigmoidectomy. *Surg Endosc,* 12(5): 448-449.

Leroy J., Milsom J. & Okuda J.(2001). *Laparoscopic sigmoidectomy for diverticulitis.* Epublication: WeBSurg.com, 1(6). Available at: http://www.websurg.com/ref/doi-ot02en165.htm

Lotze R.H. (1852). *Medicinische Psychologie und Physiologie der Seele.* Leipzig: Weidmann'sche Buchhandlung.

Miller G.A. (1956). The magical number seven plus or minus two: Some limits on our capacity for processing information. *Psychological Review,* 63: 81-97.

Milsom J.W., Böhm B. & Nakajima K. (2006). *Laparoscopic Colorectal Surgery.* New York: Springer Science + Business Media.

Nano M., Levi A.C., Borghi F., Bellora P., Bogliatto F., Garbossa D. et al. (1998). Observations on surgical anatomy for rectal cancer surgery. *Hepatogastroenterology,* 45: 717-726.

Netter F.H. (2000). *Atlas der Anatomie des Menschen.* Stuttgart, New York: Georg Thieme Verlag.

Schwandner O., Farke S., Fischer F., Eckmann C., Schiedeck T.H. & Bruch H.P. (2004). Laparoscopic colectomy for recurrent and complicated diverticulitis: a prospective study of 369 patients. *Langenbecks Arch Chir,* 389: 79-103.

Schwandner O., Farke S. & Bruch H.P. (2005). Laparoscopic colectomy for diverticulitis is not associated with increased morbitiy when compared with non-diverticular disease. *Int J Colorectal Dis,* 20: 165-172.

Schwenk W., Junghans T., Langelotz C., Haase O. & Müller J.M. (2003). *Die laparoskopische Sigmaresektion – Basistechnik, Tipps und Tricks.* Mediathek der DGCH. Available at: http://www.mediathek-dgch.de/index.cfm?9C45198EB4 C24201BA71401648D4D0F8

Schünke M., Schulte E. & Schumacher U. (2005). *Prometheus LernAtlas der Anatomie. Hals und Innere Organe.* Stuttgart, New York: Georg Thieme Verlag.

Shafik A. & Mostafa H. (1996). Study of the arterial pattern of the rectum and its clinical application. *Acta Anat,* 157: 80-86.

Sonoda T. & Milsom J.W. (2006). *Segmental Colon Resection. ACS Surgery: Principles and Practice, Gastrointestinal Tract and Abdomen.* WebMD. Available at: http://www.acssurgery.com:6200/sample/ACS0534.pdf

Steinert R., Lippert H. & Reymond M.A. (2002). Tumour cell dissemination during laparoscopy: Prevention and therapeutic opportunities. *Dig Surg,* 19: 464-472.

Tomita H., Marcello P.W. & Milsom J.W. (1999). Laparoscopic surgery of the colon and rectum. *World J Surg,* 23: 397-405.

Troidl H. (1995). Fehleranalyse – Methode zur Vermeidung von Fehlern/Komplikationen in der Chirurige. In K. Kremer, W. Platzer & H.W. Schreiber (Hrsg.), *Chirurgische Operationslehre. Minimal-invasive Chirurgie; Band 7; Teil 2* (315-323). Stuttgart, New York: Georg Thieme Verlag.

List of key words

Titles available

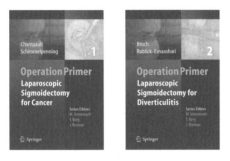

Volume 1: Laparoscopic Sigmoidectomy for Cancer   ISBN 978-3-540-78454-8

Volume 2: Laparoscopic Sigmoidectomy for Diverticulitis   ISBN 978-3-540-78451-7

Titles in preparation

Thyroidectomy with Harmonic FOCUS® shears

Laparoscopic Rectal Resection

Laparoscopic Cholecystectomy

Clipless Laparoscopic Cholecystectomy with Harmonic® shears

Laparoscopic Gastric Banding with the Swedish Adjustable Gastric Band (SAGB VC)

Stapled Transanal Rectum Resection (S.T.A.R.R.) with CONTOUR Transtar®

Open Rectal Resection